Swami Muktananda

MYSTERY *of the* MIND

Swami Muktananda

MYSTERY *of the* MIND

SIDDHA YOGA®

A SIDDHA YOGA PUBLICATION
PUBLISHED BY SYDA FOUNDATION®
www.siddhayoga.org

Published by SYDA Foundation
371 Brickman Rd., P.O. Box 600, South Fallsburg, New York 12779-0600, USA

ACKNOWLEDGMENTS
EDITORS: Peggy Bendet and Valerie Sensabaugh
PRODUCTION EDITOR: Vera Mezina
COVER DESIGN: Cheryl Crawford
SANSKRIT CONSULTANT: Elaine Fisher
COPYEDITOR: Judith Levi
TYPESETTER: Victoria Light
PRINT COORDINATOR: François Simon

Original language: Hindi

Second edition 1993

Printed in the United States of America

25 24 23 22 21 20 19 4 5 6 7 8

Library of Congress Catalog Card Number: 81-50159

ISBN 978-0-911-30751-1

ABOUT THE SYDA FOUNDATION

The SYDA Foundation is a not-for-profit organization that protects, preserves, and facilitates the dissemination of the Siddha Yoga teachings. The SYDA Foundation also guides the philanthropic expressions of the Siddha Yoga path. These include The PRASAD Project, which provides health, education, and sustainable development programs for children, families, and communities in need; and the Muktabodha Indological Research Institute, which contributes to the preservation of the scriptural heritage of India.

NOTE ON THE TEXT

Throughout the text, terms in languages other than English are printed in italics; all proper names are printed in roman type. The standard international transliteration conventions for Sanskrit and modern South Asian languages have been employed. For the reader's convenience, a Sanskrit pronunciation guide is included on pages 42-43.

Contents

The Siddha Yoga Lineage

SIDDHA YOGA is a spiritual path of teachings and practices imparted by the Siddha Yoga Gurus.

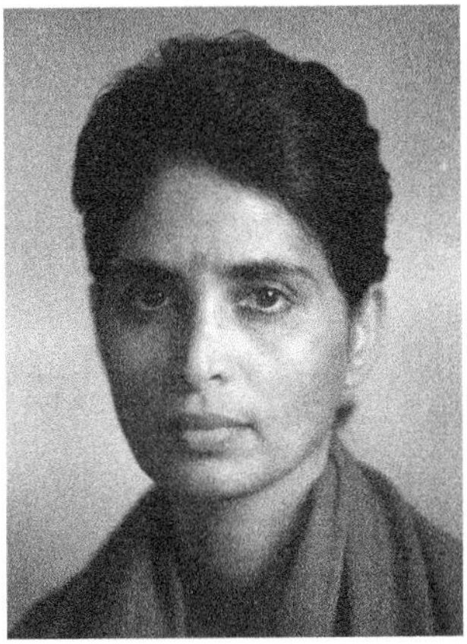

GURUMAYI CHIDVILASANANDA

GURUMAYI CHIDVILASANANDA is the Guru of the Siddha Yoga path. Gurumayi is a Siddha Guru, an enlightened meditation Master who has the rare power to awaken within a human being the inner spiritual energy known as Kuṇḍalinī Śakti. Seekers around the world have received this sacred initiation, *śaktipāt dīkṣā*, from Gurumayi and, with her guidance, progress toward the highest spiritual attainment — the unwavering experience of divinity within themselves and all of creation.

Gurumayi received the divine power and authority of the Guru of the Siddha Yoga path from her Guru, Swami Muktananda, in 1982.

SWAMI MUKTANANDA, affectionately known by his students as Baba, received *śaktipāt dīkṣā*, in 1947 from his Guru, Bhagavan Nityananda. In 1961, Bhagavan Nityananda transmitted to Baba Muktananda the power and authority to bestow *śaktipāt* initiation.

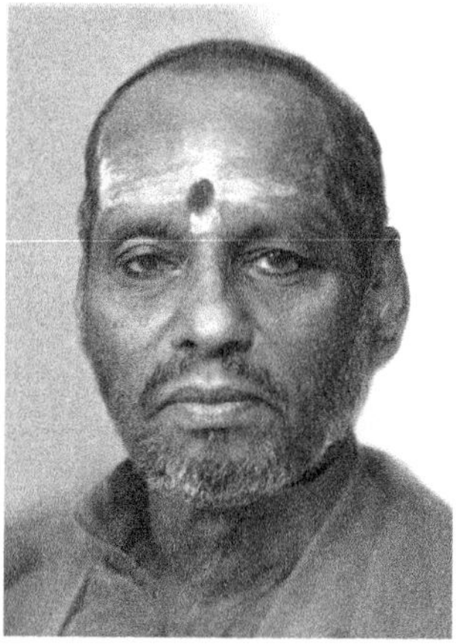

SWAMI MUKTANANDA

Baba gave form and articulation to the Siddha Yoga path, bringing together the teachings that he received from his Guru, the spiritual knowledge and practices from the timeless wisdom of India, and his own direct experience. In the course of three world tours between 1970 and 1982, Baba imparted the Siddha Yoga teachings and practices to seekers around the globe.

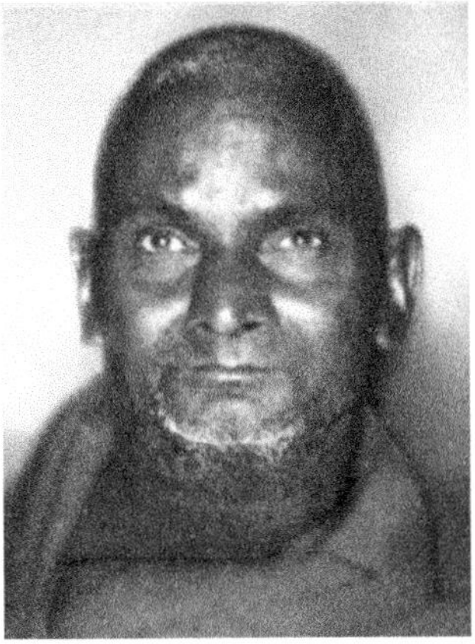

BHAGAVAN NITYANANDA

BHAGAVAN NITYANANDA, also known as Bade Baba, was a *śaktipāt* Guru and a saint widely revered throughout India. He came to settle in the village of Gaṇeśpurī in Mahārāṣṭra state. It was here, in the mid-1940s, that Swami Muktananda became a disciple of Bhagavan Nityananda. In 1956, Bhagavan Nityananda asked Swami Muktananda to establish his own Ashram less than a mile from Gaṇeśpurī. This became the Siddha Yoga Ashram known as Gurudev Siddha Peeṭh.

MYSTERY *of the* MIND

The mind is the mystery of human life. It can be the garden of joy or the secret path to death. It can show us heaven, or it can take us to hell. The mind tortures everyone — rich people and poor people, men and women, writers and scientists, politicians, businessmen, and professors. One person is unhappy because he dislikes his occupation, while another is miserable because he fears death. One person suffers because he has no wife, while another burns because his wife is beautiful and he is afraid she will be taken away from him. In the developed countries of the world, people have enough food, clothing, education, and wealth. Still, there is so much mental suffering that the number of psychiatrists and mental hospitals is constantly increasing. The fact is that a person who is not troubled by his mind is very rare.

Yet the same mind that is the cause of suffering is also the means of attaining the highest happiness. One who has truly understood the mind and has brought it under his control lives in bliss. One who has made the mind pure, strong, and still is able to accomplish anything. This is why the Indian sages have said that the mind is the cause of both happiness and unhappiness, both bondage and liberation. If there is anything worth knowing in this world, it is the mind.

In India there are many great holy books. There are four Vedas and four subsidiary Vedas, one hundred and eight Upaniṣads, eighteen Purāṇas, twenty-one Āgamas, thirty-two

Smṛtis, and six philosophical systems. These scriptures speak very little about how to attain God; instead, they are almost entirely devoted to describing means of purifying and stilling the mind. Why is the mind considered to be so significant? It is said, "Because of *manas*, the mind, we are *mānava*, human." Without it, we are nothing but God. The scriptures and the saints say that the individual soul is not a separate entity but a part of God. It is completely pure and the embodiment of supreme bliss. Thinking that we are without God is like a fish thinking that it has never seen water. A fish would have no life without water; water is the element in which it lives. We are in the same condition. Our life is in God. In God our breath moves in and out. It is God who makes our senses function and God who witnesses our very thoughts. God lives within us in the form of the inner Self, the pure I-awareness that has been with us since we came into the world. Although people superimpose different notions onto that I-consciousness — notions such as "I am a man," "I am a woman," "I am clever," "I am stupid" — it remains completely free. The inner "I," which is closer to us than our own breath, is divine. Yet people feel far from God; they think that they have not attained God. Why? Because of the delusion of the mind.

Once we know the mind, it becomes very easy to rid ourselves of that delusion. When we are suffering from a disease, we have it diagnosed, because once we discover its cause, it is easy to cure. Similarly, once we know the mind, we can easily find a remedy for its troubles. For this reason, knowledge of the mind is essential for all of us.

The IMPORTANCE *of the* MIND

The mind is the greatest of God's gifts. It is said, "In this world or any other, everything is attained through the mind." In fact, the scriptures say that the individual exists because of the mind. We have many beautiful senses and instruments in the body, but the mind is the most important of them all. It is only because of the mind that we are able to function in the world. If we lose the use of our arms and legs, we can still function. Even if we lose our eyes, we can live happily. But without the mind, we cannot function. If the mind becomes deranged, a writer cannot write, a professor cannot teach, a dancer cannot dance, a lawyer cannot practice law. If you lose the use of your mind, what is left?

Once a great industrialist came to visit my Guru. He owned a sugar mill and several factories that employed thousands of people. However, as a result of incessant thinking and worrying, his mind had ceased to function and he had to be carried around on a stretcher. His wealth and possessions were useless to him; he needed a doctor and two nurses to look after him. His body was alive, but he was as good as dead.

The fact is that if the mind is not in good condition, if it is not disciplined and restrained, then no matter what you have in this world, you will suffer. Mental disease is nothing but the state of a mind whose thoughts have gone out of control. A person may have a beautiful family, great wealth, and fame, but if his mind is not under his control, these things will bring him no satisfaction. However, if his mind is quiet and peaceful, if it allows him to sleep at night without the help of pills, then he is rich even if he possesses nothing.

Yet how are we to control the mind? The mind is not an object or a substance that can be brought under our thumb. It is all-powerful. Even if we try to repress it through meditation and yoga, it will carry us away. If we were to try to measure the mind, we would never get to the bottom of it. Jñāneśvar Mahārāj wrote, "You cannot know the ways of the mind. It is so vast that all three worlds are too small to contain its wanderings." In the *Bhagavad-gītā*, Arjuna says to the Lord:

cañcalaṃ hi manaḥ kṛṣṇa pramāthi balavad dṛḍham |
tasyāhaṃ nigrahaṃ manye vāyor iva suduṣkaram ||

O Lord, the mind is restless, fickle, turbulent, strong, and obstinate. I think that it is as difficult to control as the wind.[1]

The mind follows the pull of the senses and overpowers your discrimination. Just as a storm takes a ship here and there until it is shattered, the mind can take a person anywhere. It is the native place of fear, the birthplace of duality. It turns determination upside down and transforms courage into cowardice. At one moment it is happy, and at the next moment it is miserable. For a while it considers something to be very good, but before long it comes to think of that same thing as very bad. The mind is never satisfied. One day it is happy as you walk with a friend. The next morning it makes you telephone that friend and say, "Our relationship is finished; I don't feel like being with you anymore." In fact, all our feelings and attitudes arise from the mind. It is said, "Man is what he thinks." The Upaniṣads say:

kāmaḥ saṅkalpo vicikitsā śraddhā'śraddhā dhṛtir
adhṛtir hrīr dhīr bhīr ity etat sarvaṃ mana eva

Desire, lust, the tendency to believe and the tendency not to believe, doubt and knowledge, unity and diversity, agitation and peace, fear and courage, embarrassment and shamelessness are all the work of the mind.[2]

The great saint Sundardās writes in one of his poems, "Whether you consider something to be high or low, painful or pleasurable, honorable or dishonorable is due to the mind." Thus, it is the mind that creates your world. Gaudapāda, the Guru of the great Śaṅkarācārya, says:

yathā svapne dvayābhāsaṃ cittaṃ calati māyayā |
tathā jāgraddvayābhāsaṃ cittaṃ calati māyayā ||
advayaṃ ca dvayābhāsaṃ cittaṃ svapne na saṃśayaḥ |
advayaṃ ca dvayābhāsaṃ tathā jāgran na saṃśayaḥ ||

When you are asleep, you see different worlds of duality in your dreams. These dreams exist because of the mind. Just as the mind creates worlds in the dream state, it creates the world of duality in the waking state.[3]

Each person creates an independent world in his mind and then dwells in his creation.

Just as the world of an individual is the product of his mind, the universe is a product of the mind of the Lord. In the *Bhagavad-gītā* the Lord says that all the creatures of the world arose from his mind.[4] According to the great philosophy of Kashmir Shaivism, the universe is the sport of the mind of the supreme Lord. Shaivism says that in the beginning the Lord was alone. Then he had the thought, "Let me become many," and from his thought the world manifested. The universe is contained in the cosmic mind, and the mind of the individual is a portion of it. Therefore, the Upaniṣads say,

"Worship the mind as a great deity." In the *Bhagavad-gītā* the Lord says, *indriyāṇāṃ manaś cāsmi*, "Among the ten senses, I am the mind."[5]

MIND *and* PRĀṆA

Where does the individual mind originate? The Upaniṣads say that the mind is the pulsation of the inner Self.[6] It arises from the Self, and along with the vital force, the *prāṇa*, it permeates the entire body. The Upaniṣads also tell us that the mind is united with the vital force:

> *ātmana eṣa prāṇo jāyate* |
> *yathaiṣā puruṣe chāyaitasminn etadātatam* |
> *manokṛtenāyāty asmiñ śarīre* ||

> From the inner Consciousness originates *prāṇa*, and with the help of the mind, it moves in the body and carries out its functions.[7]

The yogic scriptures explain that *prāṇa* assumes five forms, and in these forms it sustains the body. One form of *prāṇa* is *vyāna*, which pervades every pore of the body. The mind works with the *vyāna prāṇa*, moving in the body and enabling us to experience the world through our five senses of perception and five organs of action. The mind is the commander-in-chief of all these senses. Only when the mind is connected to the senses and instruments in our system do they work for us; without the help of the mind, none of them can function. When a fly sits on your thigh, you know it is there only if your mind is paying attention. Someone may be standing directly in front of you, but you will see him only if your mind is present. All of our sensations are experienced in the mind. In this way, the mind is the source of our mundane experience. Everything that happens to us, within and without, happens because of the mind.

The mind is controlled by *prāṇa*; when the *prāṇa* stops moving, the mind becomes still. It is because the mind and *prāṇa* are united that we experience pain and pleasure. For this reason, a yogi who is able to separate the mind from the *prāṇa* goes beyond both.

I had a friend named Kavi Vināyaka, a great poet-saint. Once he developed a cancerous growth on his arm. His disciples nagged him to have it removed, until at last he agreed to have an operation. When the time came, he refused to allow the doctors to give him an anesthetic. He sat in a chair, and as the doctors worked on the cancer, he talked to his disciples. The doctors warned him not to speak, but he told them, "You do your work; I'm doing mine." While he talked to his disciples, the doctors finished the operation.

Later they asked him why he had not felt any pain. He explained, "You do not experience happiness or unhappiness because of outer circumstances. Neither fragrance nor stench can affect me if I am not aware of them. There has to be a knower to experience pain and pleasure; otherwise, who will experience them? That experiencer is the mind. While you were performing the operation, I pulled the *prāṇa* and the mind away from my arm and kept them in my heart."

This also occurs in our ordinary experience. When a doctor is about to perform an operation, he administers an anesthetic, which makes the patient's mind unconscious. In that state, the patient experiences neither happiness nor unhappiness, neither pleasure nor pain. Only when the mind is functioning do we experience these things. For this reason, the Upaniṣads tell us that heat and cold, pleasure and pain, delight and grief are the nature of the inner psychic instrument, the mind.

The MOVEMENT *of the* MIND

Indian psychologists, the great sages who expounded yoga, understood that the mind takes four forms, each with a different function. When the mind is filled with thoughts, it is called *manas*. When it contemplates, it is called *citta*.[8] When it makes decisions, it is called *buddhi*, intellect. When it takes on the feeling of "I"-ness, it is called *ahamkāra*, ego. Together, these four functions are called the *antahkarana*, or inner psychic instrument.

The Upaniṣads state that the seat of the mind is the heart. Contemporary doctors do not accept this fact, believing that the mind is located in the brain. Yet when a person undergoes a crisis, it is the heart that trembles. When we become filled with fear, we experience this sensation in the heart. There are three *nāḍīs*, or subtle channels, that lead from the heart to the *sahasrāra*, the spiritual center in the crown of the head, and that is why it seems that the mind is in the head. Nonetheless, the central abode of the mind is the heart, and if we meditate deeply, we will come to know that.

The yogic scriptures describe the heart as a lotus with eight petals. The mind is located at the stalk of that lotus. Each petal contains a different quality, and as the individual soul, along with the mind and *prāṇa*, keeps moving around the different petals of the lotus, it experiences the qualities of those petals. That is why an individual feels different at every moment of the day. For example, he may be sitting quietly, thinking about someone he loves and experiencing love. A moment later, he thinks about someone else and is suddenly filled with hostility or anger. As time passes, he becomes infatuated with something. A little while later, he becomes so upset that he feels he is going crazy. Nothing has actually happened; he has only been sitting still and thinking. The *Dhyānabindu Upaniṣad* explains this very beautifully: "When the individual soul lights on a particular petal that is directed toward the east and is white, it is filled with good feeling. When it moves toward the black petal in the south, it is filled with anger." In this way, many different feelings arise and subside in the realm of the mind.

Just as it is the nature of fire to burn, it is the nature of the mind to think and wander all the time. The mind is composed of thoughts and doubts. It constantly casts up dreams and fantasies, creating its own world and then destroying it. It builds thought castles in the air and then gets entangled in its own creation. In this way, it creates its own suffering and undergoes the consequences. Some modern psychologists believe that the mind can be satisfied if you let it run free, if you let it have whatever it wants. But this is not the case. The mind can never be satisfied in this way; it will always create a mountain of desires.

Once there was a poor man. Wherever he went, poverty followed him. One day, in his wanderings, he found himself in the abode of celestial beings where there is a heavenly garden called Nandanvān. There he sat down under a beautiful tree, which happened to be a wish-fulfilling tree. A fresh breeze was blowing, and as he sat there, the man began to feel happy. "What a beautiful garden," he thought. "What a wonderful place I have come to!"

No matter where we go, the mind goes with us. We can never leave it behind, and it never leaves us alone. Even though this man was sitting in such a beautiful place, he could not sit quietly. Instead, he began to think. "If only I had a girlfriend with me, how much more I would enjoy myself." This was a wish-fulfilling tree, so the moment he thought of a girlfriend, a beautiful girl came sashaying up to him. He greeted her with pleasure. Now there were two of them sitting under the wish-fulfilling tree. For a little while the man was happy, but then once again he began to think. "If only we had a beautiful house with two bedrooms and luxurious furniture," he said to himself. Immediately, an attractive modern bungalow appeared, filled with everything they could need. The man and his girlfriend walked inside. He thought, "This is great, but now we need servants and a cook. We should have a gourmet meal to eat!" As soon as he had this thought, some servants appeared and prepared a meal. They set it on the table, and the man and his girlfriend sat down. The table was spread with delicious dishes. The man took a spoonful of food and was just about to taste it when he had another thought. (This is the nature of the mind — it always doubts.) "What's going on?" he wondered. "I thought of a girl, and a girl appeared. I thought of a house, and a house materialized. I thought of all these dishes, and even they manifested. This must be the work of a demon!" Immediately, a demon stood before him with its mouth wide open. "Alas, he's going to eat me up!" the man cried. And the demon ate him up.

This man was sitting under a wish-fulfilling tree. He could have thought of anything, but instead he thought of a demon. We are all in the same predicament. Instead of thinking good thoughts, instead of thinking of ourselves as noble, great, and sublime, we constantly think of ourselves as insignificant creatures, and thus we become petty and small.

Thought has infinite power. That is why the sages pray, "O my mind, always think well of yourself and others." When your mind is restless and turbulent, when you think negatively all the time, you harm not only yourself, but others as well. A good man, by continually thinking "I am a sinner, I am a sinner," will end up being a sinner, while a bad man, by continually thinking "I am pure, I am sublime," will end up being pure. It is our thoughts that create our heaven and hell; by our thoughts, we can make ourselves experience divinity or we can put ourselves down until we feel like hellish insects. Therefore, it is of the highest importance that we think positively about ourselves and other people.

We are constantly eating the products of our thoughts. Once a poor man was sitting under a tree. For several days, he had had nothing to eat, and his stomach was beginning to give him trouble. In order to satisfy it, he began to cook in his imagination. First he cooked a rice dish, and then a vegetable and some soup. After he had finished cooking, he started to eat. He ate the soup and the rice, and then he ate the vegetable. But he had put too many chilies in the vegetable, and they burned his mouth. He began to fan his mouth, crying, "Oooh, oooh!" Another man was sitting under a nearby tree, and when he saw this peculiar behavior, he called out, "Hey, brother, what's the matter with you?"

"I cooked some vegetables in my imagination, and I accidently put in too many chilies!"

"You fool," said the second man. "Why did you put in so many chilies? Since you were only cooking in your imagination, couldn't you have made ice cream?"

In the same way, if we could train the mind to think positive thoughts, then it would become very pure and very strong. But because of our present mental weakness, we let the mind wander here and there. In that way, we continually burn in the mind's creations.

It is the mind that makes us perceive this universe as being filled with diversity. God created the universe in one way, but the mind makes us see it differently. It erases God's creation, replaces it with its own, and shows us duality in God's unity. The teaching of the Upaniṣads and all the saints is *ayam ātma brahma*, "The inner Self of a human being is God."[9] There is no difference between the Self and God, but because of the mind, the Self appears to be the limited enjoyer of the senses. Actually, the Self does not experience anything, but through the mind it mingles with the senses and takes on two aspects. Mingling with the senses of perception, it makes us feel that we are the experiencer. Mingling with the organs of action, it makes us feel that we are the doer. Thus, it is the mind that is responsible for our feeling of limited agency, our feeling of imperfection.

But if the mind were to become pure, to discard all its thoughts and doubts, it would experience God everywhere. The mind, which is the cause of all suffering, would become our greatest friend. The Upaniṣads say that God immediately reveals himself to one whose mind has become pure. In fact, mental purity is not only for great beings or for those who want to attain liberation. It is necessary for people in every field, because if the mind is impure, you cannot understand things correctly. If a doctor's mind is impure, he cannot correctly diagnose a disease. But if his mind is strong and stable, he can even cure his patients through the power of his mind. Psychotherapists and psychologists particularly need to strengthen their minds. A psychotherapist spends many hours a day talking to mentally disturbed people, and if his mind is weak, he is affected by their state. He does not realize that this is happening, but over the years the effects accumulate, and he may begin to experience mental suffering.

Through spiritual practices, you can purify and strengthen

the mind. In Jñāneśvar's commentary on the *Bhagavad-gītā* — *Jñāneśvarī* — Lord Kṛṣṇa says, "If you purify your mind with thoughts of the Lord, with contemplation of the Lord, with repetition of the name of the Lord, you discover a new creation of the Lord within yourself." The mind is often compared to a mirror. If a mirror is dirty, it cannot reflect objects clearly. In the same way, a mind that has become dirty by association with outer objects cannot reflect the inner Consciousness. But if it is cleaned by the practice of spiritual discipline, you can see the Self reflected in it.

God is very close to the mind. In Kashmir Shaivism it is said, *svacchātmā sphurati satataṃ cetasi śivaḥ*, "That is supremely pure and independent, and can be experienced throbbing constantly within the mind." Pulsating within the mind, the Self makes the mind think. In fact, the Self is manifest in all our thoughts and feelings, and it is the Self that allows us to perceive everything. According to Kashmir Shaivism, the Self has two aspects: *prakāśa*, light, and *vimarśa*, understanding. *Prakāśa* illuminates everything in this world. *Vimarśa* understands that which is illumined. Through *prakāśa*, we are able to see an object. Through *vimarśa*, we are able to identify it; we are able to understand, for example, that one thing is a book and that another is a pen.

The same Self that knows the outer world is also the Knower of our thoughts and feelings. Once King Janaka asked the great sage Yājñavalkya, "Where can I find God?" Yājñavalkya replied, "God is the Witness of the mind." When the mind is full of thoughts and doubts, the inner Knower, *prakāśa* and *vimarśa*, perceives and identifies them. No matter how bad or how good we feel, that Knower remains detached from all our surges of feeling. At night, we leave the waking state and enter the state of sleep. But even when we go to sleep, that Knower within us does not sleep but remains awake and reports to us on our dreams. That inner Knower is the Self. It lives within the mind, yet remains different from the mind. The Upaniṣads say that the mind is nothing but the form, the body, of the Self. The mind cannot recognize the Self because it is its body. But when the outward-flowing mind is turned inward, it merges in its source, and you immediately experience your divinity. When the mind begins to reflect the inner Consciousness, it takes on the attributes of Consciousness. In fact, the mind that is alive, strong, and one-pointed, that has become one with the inner Self, has the same power as the Self. It is not different from the Self. For this reason, in *Jñāneśvarī* the Lord says, "O Arjuna, do not become entangled in the creation of your mind. Bring your mind under your control. Make your mind very strong and make it move in me."

YOGA, PATAÑJALI, *and the* MIND

In order to make the mind strong, we have to practice yoga. We should not think that yoga is difficult or strange, for the truth is that our lives are the embodiment of yoga. We all sit in a particular posture, and that is yoga. Our breath moves in and out, and that is *prāṇāyāma*, which is part of yoga. In order to drive a car, cook a meal, or even contemplate our beloved, we have to meditate one-pointedly. That is yoga. So we are already following some aspects of yoga in our lives. We are simply not aware of it.

In India the authoritative treatise on yoga is the *Yoga-sūtra* of Mahārṣi Patañjali. Patañjali was a great sage. He thoroughly understood the mind and brought it under his control. Only when he had come to know the Truth completely did he compose the *Yoga-sūtra*. The *Yoga-sūtra* is not a religious work but is genuine psychology. Beings like Patañjali are true psychologists, because only one who has become established in the Truth can understand how the mind works. In his *Yoga-sūtra*, Patañjali explains what the mind is, how it troubles us, what we can do to control it, and the state of beings who have controlled their minds.

In the second *sūtra*, Patañjali describes yoga: *yogaś citta-vṛtti-nirodhaḥ*, "Yoga is the stilling of the *vṛttis* [modifications] of the mind."[10] He does not say that the purpose of yoga is to still the mind or to eradicate it. As we have already seen, the mind is a pulsation of God, a ray of the Self. It can never be destroyed. It is not the mind that tortures us. We are tortured by the *vṛttis*, the waves of thoughts and feelings that cause the mind to become agitated. It is these that must be stilled if we are to experience the Self.

Patañjali explains that the mind has five kinds of *vṛttis*. Some are painful and some are nonpainful. The painful modifications arise from ignorance, unhappiness, turmoil, and the continual outward movement of the mind. The nonpainful modifications arise when the mind turns within and, in meditation, becomes one with the Self.

The *vṛttis* of the mind are right knowledge (*pramāṇa*), wrong knowledge (*viparyaya*), fantasy (*vikalpa*), sleep (*nidrā*), and memory (*smṛti*). *Pramāṇa* has three subdivisions: *pratyakṣa*, *anumāna*, and *āgama pramāṇa*.

Pratyakṣa pramāṇa is the right knowledge that is received through direct perception. If I see someone in front of me, I know from direct experience whether that person is a man or a woman. In the same way, when you turn inside and meditate for a long time, it is through direct perception that you eventually realize the Truth within. Then you are confident of the existence of the Truth, because you see it directly. When the great Sūfī saint Hazrat Bāyazīd Bistāmī was in meditation and began to declare "I am God," his statement was the result of *pratyakṣa*, direct perception.

The second kind of right knowledge is indirect knowledge, or *anumāna pramāṇa*, in which one knows the Truth by deduction or inference. For example, if you see smoke on a mountainside, you infer that there must be a fire there, because you know from experience that smoke comes from fire. In the same way, when we see lights within during meditation, we infer that these are the lights of the inner worlds.

The third kind of correct knowledge is *āgama pramāṇa*.

Āgama means scriptures, so this is the knowledge derived from scriptural texts and from the testimony of great beings. During my *sādhanā* of meditation, I perceived the lights of the four bodies, one inside the other.[11] I saw their qualities and colors, but I did not come to the conclusion that they were my bodies. Then I began to read the scriptures, the authoritative books. I read the poems of Jñāneśvar Mahārāj, Tukārām Mahārāj, and Kabīr, as well as some of the Upaniṣads, and there I found these four bodies, along with their colors and qualities, very well explained. In this way, *āgama pramāṇa* confirmed my experience.

The second major modification of the mind is *viparyaya vṛtti*. *Viparyaya* means wrong knowledge. Patañjali says, *viparyayo mithyā-jñānam atad-rūpa-pratiṣṭham*, "Wrong knowledge is a false conception of something whose real form does not correspond to such a conception."[12] This *vṛtti* makes you believe that the Self is a man or a woman. It makes a person who is going to live for a long time keep thinking, "I am going to die." It makes you doubt your beloved, wondering whether he or she has the same feelings as before. In Vedānta, *viparyaya* is explained by the analogy of a person who sees a rope and screams in fear, thinking it is a snake. Psychologists must be very aware of *viparyaya*, since it is this *vṛtti* that makes a healthy person feel he is diseased and turns a person with a good mind into a mental case. *Viparyaya* is the worst of all the *vṛttis*.

The third modification is *vikalpa vṛtti*. *Vikalpa* means imagination or fantasy. Patañjali says, *śabda-jñānānupātī vastu-śūnyo vikalpaḥ*, "An image conjured up by words without any substance behind them is imagination."[13] Imagination is the supporter of wrong knowledge. For example, a person may be walking down a road and come across a pillar. His imagination may say that the pillar is a thief and make him afraid. Every day I say, "God is inside you." But when people hear me, their imagination tells them, "How can God be inside me when I am in this state?" This is the imagination.

The fourth modification is *nidrā*, which means sleep. According to Patañjali, *abhāva-pratyayālambanā vṛttir nidrā*, "Sleep is the modification based on the absence of any content in the mind."[14] The *nidrā vṛtti* consists of ignorance or lack of knowledge of true Reality. It is because of this *vṛtti* that the great beings say to us, "O dear one, wake up. You have been sleeping for such a long time." This *vṛtti* does not operate only during the sleep state. Suppose that I am lecturing about a high principle. There may be a person present whose eyes are open and who appears to be listening, but who is not taking in what I am saying. This is also a manifestation of the *vṛtti* of sleep.

The fifth modification is *smṛti*, or memory. *Anubhūta-viṣayāsampramoṣaḥ smṛtiḥ*, "Memory is nothing but the impressions of the other four modifications, which are not allowed to escape."[15] A person may be sitting in meditation and suddenly remember that twelve years ago he had a fight with someone. Immediately, he will be in agony. Sometimes a person will tell me, "My girlfriend left me." I will reply, "Very good; forget her." But the person will say, "I can't. I constantly remember her, and the memory disturbs me." Memory is the secretary of the other four *vṛttis*; no matter where you are, it opens the file and shows you what took place in the past.

So we are tortured not by the mind, but by the five modifications of the mind. All afflictions are created by these modifications. As long as they do not become quiet, we act according to the feelings of the mind; we do everything according to our mental tendencies. This is why we experience pain. Truly speaking, there is no suffering in God's creation; suffering occurs only when we act according to the *vṛttis* of the mind.

Therefore, Patañjali says, "Try to still the modifications of the mind." How can they be stilled? *Abhyāsa-vairāgyābhyāṃ tan-nirodhaḥ*, "By intense practice and by detachment, they can be stilled."[16] All five modifications of the mind can be brought under control by these two means: practice and detachment. (However, you must practice ceaselessly, since for so many years you have been practicing the five modifications of the mind.) There are many spiritual practices, but the best is the awareness of your identity with the Truth — the constant remembrance of *So'ham*, the awareness of "I am That." Similarly, true detachment is the renunciation of your sense of duality, your various concepts such as "I am a man," "I am a woman," "I am a sinner," or "I am upset." As you practice the awareness of unity for a long time with devotion and reverence, you become grounded in the true nature of the Self. Then the five modifications of the mind become quiet.

Not everyone's mind is strong enough to maintain the constant awareness of unity. For this reason, Patañjali gives various practices that are suitable for different seekers. One of the greatest of these is mantra repetition. A mantra is a cosmic word or sound vibration. In fact, mantra is the vibration of the Self. It is the true speech of the Self, which arises from within. In mundane life, a word is one with the object it denotes, and it helps to put us in touch with that object. Similarly, the mantra, which is the name of God, is one with God and very easily puts us in touch with the God within. The scriptures say, *mantra maheśvaraḥ*, "Mantra is God." There is no difference between God and his name. Mantra has all the powers of God. Above all, it has the power to purify the mind and bring it to the Self.

It is very important, however, that you repeat a mantra with the awareness that the goal of the mantra is your own Self. If someone abuses us, the words affect us immediately. This is because we identify ourselves with them; we believe ourselves to be the object of those words. In the same way, when we repeat the mantra, we should identify ourselves as its object. We should remember that there is no difference between ourselves, the mantra, and the goal of the mantra. As we repeat the mantra with this awareness, the mind gradually merges into the mantra and becomes one with the Self.

CONCENTRATION

Patañjali's main technique for making the mind strong and one-pointed is concentration, or *dhāraṇā*. The mind is troubled because it constantly thinks of different objects. In order to still the mind, Patañjali recommends that we choose a particular object and focus the mind one-pointedly on that.

There are many objects for concentration. The yogic scriptures recommend focusing on the space between the eyebrows. The *Bhagavad-gītā* recommends watching the tip of the nose. In the book *I Am That*, I recommend watching the space between the breaths, the space where the mantra *So'ham* dissolves. You can focus on the heart, the navel, or the base of the spine. However, the best object of meditation is the Self, or the *So'ham* mantra, which is the mantra of the Self. It is the nature of the mind to become whatever it dwells upon; this is also its glory. Whatever the mind contemplates is what you become. In *Tantrāloka*, a great work of Kashmir Shaivism, it is said, "An embodied individual soul becomes completely immersed in that upon which he focuses his mind." The sages compare the mind to water; whatever color you put into it is the color it becomes. When the mind lights on an object, it becomes one with that object. A poem by the great saint Sundardās describes the mind's tendency to take on the qualities of whatever it thinks about:

> The mind that constantly thinks of women
> becomes effeminate.
> The mind that dwells on anger burns in the fire of anger.

The mind that is immersed in *māyā* (illusion)
falls into the well of illusion.
The mind that always contemplates the Absolute
becomes the Absolute.

For this reason, one who wants to experience the Self should make the mind contemplate the Self. Just as the mind becomes one with objects on the outside, when it turns within and contemplates Consciousness, it imbibes the qualities of Consciousness and becomes supremely blissful.

Because the mind has this tendency to take on the qualities of whatever it focuses upon, Patañjali recommends another, particularly easy means of stilling and purifying the mind: *vīta-rāga-viṣayaṃ vā cittam*, "Focus the mind on a being who has risen above passion and attachment."[17] Such a great being has become one with the Self. His mind has become mindless; it has become the Self. When you make such a being the object of your thoughts, then your mind, like his, becomes free of thoughts. I used to sit before my Guru for two or three hours at a time. I would fix my mind on him, and as I did so, my mind would become quiet. It would become mindless; it would become just like him.

This state of stillness is called *nirvikalpa*, or the thought-free state. It is a state of great joy. Unhappiness is nothing but the net of thoughts, and when you go beyond thoughts, you experience bliss. In that state, the mind becomes one with the Self and imbibes its power. Do not think that if the mind becomes still, it will become useless and you will be unable to function. The more still and one-pointed the mind becomes, the more work it is able to do. If someone dams a stream and stops its flow, that stream becomes a lake with enough water to satisfy the thirst of thousands of people. In the same way, when the flow of the mind is controlled, it can accomplish anything. A psychologist who has brought his mind under control can cure mental patients through its power, just by sitting in a room with them. Through the power of the mind, great beings can awaken the spiritual energy in others. Through the power of their concentrated minds, the ancient sages were able to bring about a new creation. Through the power of feeling that arises in the mind, you can turn an enemy into a friend; you can even turn poison into nectar.

The great saint Mīrābāī was a queen in Rājasthān, India. She was always immersed in love for God. She used to wear anklets and dance while singing God's name, and for her, nothing was different from him. But her husband, the king, thought that by her devotion she was bringing disgrace to the family name and decided to have her poisoned. When Mīrābāī was given the poison, she drank it with the awareness that it was God, and so it did not affect her. This was the result of the sublime feeling of her mind. It was not a great miracle, for through meditation a person should be able to make his mind so strong that even if an atomic bomb were to explode near him, it would not affect him.

The POWER *of the* MIND

Innumerable powers come to a person whose mind is controlled. For example, he gains knowledge of the future. His mind becomes so subtle that it can enter others' minds and hearts and know what is taking place there. Once the great saint Tukārām Mahārāj went to visit another saint, Samārth Rāmdās. Rāmdās was the Guru of the well-known and popular king Śivājī, who had conquered many states and was about to be crowned sovereign. Tukārām arrived a few days before Śivājī's coronation. Rāmdās was sitting very still, completely absorbed in the thought of the horse he was going to buy and decorate for Śivājī to ride during the ceremony. Tukārām waited quietly until Rāmdās emerged from his state of absorption. When Rāmdās opened his eyes and saw Tukārām, he asked, "Tukārām, when did you come?"

"I came while you were buying the horse for Śivājī," Tukārām replied.

Such powers are commonplace for a being whose mind is under control. In fact, you do not have to be a great yogi to have them. In Russia there lived a man named Wolf Messing, who was very well known for the unique and strange power of his mind. On one occasion, in order to test his mental power, Premier Stalin told Messing to go to one of the government banks and, with the power of his mind, to steal 100,000 rubles. Messing went into the bank, walked up to a teller, and handed him a piece of paper torn from a school notebook. Then he told him telepathically to hand over 100,000 rubles. The teller took the piece of paper, reached inside a drawer, and gave Messing the money.

I relate this story not so you will go out and rob a bank, but to demonstrate the power of the mind. In the *Yoga-sūtra*, Patañjali also explains the technique for acquiring *siddhis*. If one meditates on an object for a long time, that object eventually disappears; the seer and the seen merge into each other. When the seer and the seen and the process of seeing become one, your practice of meditation culminates, and you gain mastery over that object. If you practice this technique constantly and uninterruptedly, you gain *sāmyama śakti*, the power of concentration, through which one acquires mastery over the elements. If such a person performs *sāmyama* on an elephant, he gains the strength of an elephant. By focusing his attention on the sun, by bringing its power into himself, he can see what is taking place in the entire solar system. By doing *sāmyama* on the throat region, he can acquire the power to do without food or drink. Once Muktābāī, the sister of Jñāneśvar Mahārāj, wanted to make *puraṇ-polis*, sweet pancakes, but no one would give her a pan. So Jñāneśvar lay down on the ground and performed *sāmyama* on fire. In this way, he made his back so hot that Muktābāī was able to cook *puraṇ-polis* on his back. Such powers come automatically to a being who is immersed in God. They do not have much importance, nor do they bring you closer to God. I describe them here only to demonstrate what the mind can do.

The MIND *as* CONSCIOUSNESS

Still, the question remains: what is the real nature of the mind? To understand this, we have to look at the mind from the viewpoint of Kashmir Shaivism. In the texts of Kashmir Shaivism, it is said that the mind is itself supreme Consciousness. Shaivism describes the mind as the radiance of *cit-śakti*, the power of God. *Cit-śakti* is the creative energy of the supreme Being. It is the conscious power that creates the universe in supreme freedom, manifesting all the diverse shapes and forms of this cosmos within its own being.

As it becomes this universe, universal Consciousness voluntarily contracts itself and accepts limitations, and then it is called the mind. The *Pratyabhijñā-hṛdayam*, one of the principal texts of Kashmir Shaivism, states, *citir eva cetana-padād avarūḍhā cetya-saṅkocinī cittam*, "When universal Consciousness, *citi*, descends from its lofty status as pure Consciousness and assumes the form of different objects, it becomes *citta*, the individual consciousness, or mind, by contracting itself in accordance with the objects perceived."[18] So the mind is nothing but Consciousness in a contracted form. That Consciousness is one with the Self, so the mind is simply that aspect of the Self which has taken the form of outer objects. It is just as if a sophisticated and well-dressed person were walking down a road and fell into a sewer. His clean clothes would become filthy, but beneath the dirt, he would be the same person as before. In the same way, when the universal

Consciousness becomes the mind, even in its contracted form it retains its nature as Consciousness. Just as Consciousness creates infinite outer worlds, when Consciousness becomes the mind, it continually gives birth to new universes. It creates different mental worlds, sustains them for a while, and then dissolves them within its own being. This process goes on and on. But if *citta* separates itself from outer objects and turns inside, it once again becomes *citi*, pure Consciousness. This is the true greatness and power of the mind. When this is the case, it is no wonder that the mind cannot be suppressed or controlled by force. Only through understanding and knowledge can the mind be stilled.

MĀTṚKĀ-ŚAKTI

Just as Patañjali explains how the modifications of the mind are responsible for our contracted condition, Shaivism describes the nature of the force that gives rise to these modifications. In the *Śiva-sūtra* there is an aphorism: *jñānādhiṣṭhānaṃ mātṛkā*, "It is *mātṛkā*, the uncomprehended mother, or power of sound inherent in the alphabet, that is the basis of limited knowledge."[19] When *citi* subjects itself to limitations, it manifests in the form of *mātṛkā*. *Mātṛkā-śakti* is the force behind the mind. *Mātṛkā* literally means "letters"; in Sanskrit, the letters of the alphabet are called *mātṛkās*. *Mātṛkā-śakti*, the power behind the letters, is the force that creates words, and words are responsible for our experience of limitation.

Mātṛkā arises from the deepest level of speech. Just as we have four bodies, we also have four levels of speech. The deepest level is *parā-vāk*, the cosmic tongue or supreme level of speech. This is the level of pure Consciousness. Although *parā-vāk* is all-pervasive, in the human body it is located in the region of the navel. At this level, *śakti* is absolutely pure. From here, the *śakti* rises to the *paśyantī* level, which exists in the inner heart. Here, the letters begin to take shape, but in a concealed form. Next, speech rises to the *madhyamā* level, which is located in the region of the throat. Here, the words are formed but are not yet ready to be articulated. Finally, speech rises to the *vaikharī*, or gross, level — the level of the tongue. Here, words come bursting forth in the form of verbal speech.

In *parā-vāk*, the *śakti* exists in its original, expanded state. However, when it rises to the *madhyamā* level, it becomes contracted, because it is in *madhyamā* that letters are combined. When letters first arise, they are simply sounds. But through the power of the *mātṛkā-śakti* they come together to form words, and then they begin to affect us. Letters form words; words form sentences. Each word has its own meaning, and the meaning has its own goal. By themselves, the letters *f*, *o*, *o*, *l* do not mean anything. But when they are combined, they form the word *fool*. That word has a meaning, and when you hear it, an image is carved out in the mind. When you identify with the image, it gives rise to a certain feeling, and because of that feeling you experience pain. This is how the *mātṛkā-śakti* works in the inner and outer worlds. It creates images on the screen of the mind, and these images create either joy or sorrow. Thus, the *mātṛkā-śakti*, the power of letters, creates all the different feelings and emotions that make our minds agitated.

If no letters arise in the mind, it remains still. We know this from experience. When we wake up in the morning, there is a moment or two when the mind is serene and free of thought; we are in the state of the pure "I." Then the *mātṛkā-śakti* starts to work. Words arise in the mind. We think about where we are; we think about having our tea; we think about brushing our teeth. In this way, the world comes into existence for us.

Only because of the letters can we carry on our dealings in the mundane world. Neither language nor terminology nor novels nor scriptures exist apart from *mātṛkā-śakti*. That *śakti* contains everything: desire, greed, love, purity, and impurity. Everything that happens in this world happens because of the *mātṛkā-śakti*.

Shaivism refers to three innate impurities (*malas*) that cause our understanding to become contracted. The first of these is *āṇava mala*, which makes us feel imperfect. The second is *māyīya mala*, which makes us feel that we are different from others. The third is *karma mala*, which makes us feel that we are the doer of our good and bad actions. The knowledge arising from these impurities binds us and makes us believe that we are limited, petty creatures. The basis of these impurities is the ideas and concepts arising from words, and the source of all these words is the *mātṛkā-śakti*. Through the *mātṛkā-śakti*, we experience contracted feelings like "I am imperfect," "I am a psychologist," "Nobody likes me," or "I have more understanding than anyone else." Through the work of the *mātṛkā*, waves of thought and imagination keep arising and subsiding; infinite thoughts are born and die.

Once there was a poor laborer named Sheikh Mahmūd. One day his employer gave him a clay pot full of ghee (clarified butter) and told him to carry it to the next town. "If you do this," the employer said, "I will give you two rupees. If you drop the pot, you will have to pay for the ghee."

Sheikh Mahmūd put the pot on his head and set out along the road. As he was walking, he started to think, "I'm going to get two rupees. What shall I do with them?" In those days, everything was very cheap. For one rupee, you could buy twenty-five chickens. Sheikh Mahmūd said, "That's it, I'll buy chickens. They will multiply, and soon I'll have one hundred chickens, five hundred chickens, one thousand chickens, ten thousand chickens. Then I'll sell all the chickens and buy goats. I'll have goats and sheep and a big farm. The goats and sheep will multiply, and when I sell them, I'll buy goods. I'll become a big merchant. Then I'll get married and have a house. I'll go to an office, and I'll return home for lunch. I'll have a very good cook to make delicious dishes. But if the cook doesn't bring the food on time, I'll get angry and slap his face.

After all, I'll be a big merchant." As he thought about slapping the cook's face, he raised his arm. As soon as he did so, the pot of ghee went flying to the ground.

So the ghee did not reach the next town. Mahmūd did not get his two rupees. He did not buy chickens. He did not buy goats and sheep. He did not get married. He did not have a house. He did not go to an office. Nor did he slap anyone. He sat down and put his head in his hands. After a while he returned to his employer and confessed, "Master, I spilled the ghee."

The employer replied, "How could you do such a stupid thing? You've lost my week's profit!"

"O Master," said Mahmūd, "you lost a week's profit, but I lost my chickens, my goats, my house, my wife, my office, and my cook!"

This is the play of the mind. This is the power of the *mātṛkā-śakti*. One thought leads to another thought, and that thought leads to a third. The progeny of the *mātṛkā-śakti* are infinite. The *mātṛkā-śakti* keeps creating letters, and we keep experiencing them. We become infatuated with them, we identify with them, and, in this way, we become bound. Different feelings arise in the heart, and the soul keeps moving among them, experiencing pain and pleasure. The *mātṛkā-śakti* makes us forget that we are the Self. Instead of letting us experience God in everyone, it makes us feel separate from everyone. It veils our true nature and shows its own manifestations to us. The *mātṛkā-śakti* never takes a vacation, it never goes to sleep, it is never late for work, and it never retires. It dies only when we attain the thought-free state, the state of *nirvikalpa samādhi*.

Yet when it is properly understood, the *mātṛkā-śakti* also helps us to progress. It is through the *mātṛkā* that we are able to repeat the mantra and contemplate the Self. Yogis who understand the nature of *mātṛkā* pursue and watch it. They turn bad thoughts into good thoughts, making their minds steady and thus bringing the *mātṛkā* under their control. By thinking "I am the Self, I am Śiva," they use the *mātṛkā-śakti* to expand themselves. When you understand what the *mātṛkā-śakti* is, when you continually contemplate the *mātṛkā-śakti*, when you turn the mind within and make it merge in its source, then you rise above pain and pleasure. You no longer have to dance according to the whim of the *mātṛkā-śakti*.

When the mind becomes free of thoughts, it gives you bliss. At the root of the *mātṛkā-śakti* is pure knowledge. When you know the mind thoroughly, you know God, because God is at the source of the mind. Wherever the mind goes, within or without, whatever thoughts or mental constructs it experiences, whether painful or pleasurable, Consciousness is the basis for that movement. The sage Vasuguptācārya says that no matter where the mind goes, no matter what the mind thinks, Śiva, universal Consciousness, is there. When this is the case, where can the mind go to leave him behind? Just as the same clay makes infinite pots, the same Consciousness, the same *śakti* has become infinite thoughts. With this understanding, contemplate the *mātṛkā-śakti*. Watch your thoughts without becoming entangled in them. Watch how the *mātṛkā-śakti* plays, how it gives rise to letters, how the letters constitute words, how the words have their own meaning. Watch how the words create images, and how the images affect you. Watch how the infinite thoughts are born and die. This is true psychology, true knowledge of the mind.

Sit very quietly. Focus on the source of all your thoughts. With understanding and contemplation, still the mind in its source. Perceive the space where the thoughts merge and where they arise. Perceive the formless Witness at the root of the mind. Understand it and become established in it. Whenever a thought arises, cut it off. With the sword of the thought-free state, slash the noose of the mind. The great being Gaudapāda said:

> *mano-dṛśyam idaṃ dvaitaṃ yatkiñcit sacarācaram |*
> *manaso hy amanībhāve dvaitaṃ naivopalabhyate ||*

> This world, with all its animate beings and inanimate objects, is nothing but the creation of the mind. When the activities of the mind cease, there is no world, no duality.[20]

There is only God.

The INNER ENERGY

Within every human being dwells a great and divine energy, which in the language of the scriptures is called *kuṇḍalinī śakti*. The specific abode of this energy is in the center of the body, at the base of the spine. However, its power permeates our entire being and makes it possible for us to perform all our external functions. This energy has two aspects: internal and external. The outer aspect of *kuṇḍalinī* is the power that makes the heart beat, that enlivens the senses, and that makes the breath come in and go out; it is the power that allows us to function in the world. But the inner, spiritual aspect of *kuṇḍalinī* is dormant. If, through meditation, you awaken that inner energy, the mind very naturally turns inward and comes under your control.

Although the yogic scriptures describe different means of awakening this energy, it is awakened most easily through contact with a being whose energy is already fully unfolded. Such a being is called a Guru. He lives in a state of Self-realization and, by virtue of that state, has the power to awaken the *śakti* in others. Through a look, a mantra, a touch, or even a thought, he transmits his *śakti* to the people around him. When a person is in the company of someone who has a cold, the germs of the cold pass into him and he easily catches the cold. In the same way, when a person contacts a great being whose *śakti* has unfolded, the germs of *śakti* easily pass into that person and awaken his own inner *śakti*. Once that energy is awakened, yoga takes place spontaneously within, and meditation occurs on its own. This energy contains the knowledge of all the different planes of existence, and when it begins to unfold, you begin to experience the inner worlds.

The inner universe is much greater than the outer universe. Inside us are exquisite tastes and fragrances, and divine sounds, compared to which the outer music is insipid. Inside us is a divine joy, beside which the joy we experience in the outer world is merely a shadow. Inside us is a divine flame, the light of the Self, and when your inner *śakti* is awakened through meditation, you will see this light shimmering within. Perceiving this light, a great saint of India exclaimed, "I am the flame of the Lord! I am the Absolute." When you experience its blissful effulgence, you will understand that what he said is true. As you watch this divine light, your mind will become still; effortlessly, it will become established in the inner center of Consciousness.

As you meditate more and more, one day this light will explode, and you will see it everywhere. You will see the entire universe existing within it. The divine light of Consciousness will begin to fill your eyes, and then wherever you look you will see it. You will see its radiance in people, in trees, in rocks, and in buildings. You will see the same Consciousness rising and falling in every wave of thought and feeling that passes through your mind; wherever your mind goes you will find your own inner Consciousness, the creator of the world. You will see that the entire universe is contained within your own Self. You will know that everything — all the infinite modifications of the world — is nothing but your own play. You will realize that it is you who are being reflected everywhere and that it is your own reflection that passes before you all the time.

Just as a flame does not flicker where there is no wind, a

mind that has become immersed in the Self always remains blissful in the Self. A great Sūfī saint said, "My heart has become as pure as a mirror. No matter where I look, I see the image of Muhammad reflected there. Everyone is cast from the same mold. Everyone is the image of God. In all faces, I see only his face." This is the Truth. This is the teaching of the scriptures. This is the wisdom of the great beings. To know this is the purpose of human life. My Guru, Bhagavan Nityananda, used to say, "As long as the mind is alive, you are a human being. When the mind becomes mindless, you become God." This is why you must turn the mind within and make it still: so you can know the great divinity that exists within you and live in ecstasy.

Notes

1. *Bhagavad-gītā*, 6.34.
2. *Bṛhadāraṇyaka Upaniṣad*, 1.5.3.
3. Gaudapāda, *Gaudapāda Kārikā*, 4.61-62.
4. *Bhagavad-gītā*, 10.6.
5. *Bhagavad-gītā*, 10.22.
6. *Muṇḍaka Upaniṣad*, 2.1.3: "From him are born life, mind, and senses."
7. *Praśna Upaniṣad*, 3.3.
8. *Citta* literally means "mind-stuff." It is the unconscious mind, the great storehouse that we draw on for contemplation.
9. *Māṇḍūkya Upaniṣad*, 1.2.
10. Patañjali's *Yoga-sūtra*, 1.2.
11. According to Vedantic philosophy, the human spirit is encased in four bodies. These are the gross body, in which we experience the waking state; the subtle body, in which we dream; the causal body, into which we retire during deep sleep; and the supracausal body, which is the body of the superconscious state of meditation.
12. Patañjali's *Yoga-sūtra*, 1.8.
13. *Yoga-sūtra*, 1.9.
14. *Yoga-sūtra*, 1.10.
15. *Yoga-sūtra*, 1.11.
16. *Yoga-sūtra*, 1.12.
17. *Yoga-sūtra*, 1.37.
18. *Pratyabhijñā-hṛdayam*, sutra 5.
19. *Śiva-sūtra*, 1.4.
20. Gaudapāda, *Gaudapāda Kārikā*, 3.31.

Guide to Sanskrit Pronunciation

In Sanskrit every letter is pronounced; there are no silent letters. Every letter has only one sound, except for the letter **v** (see below).

LENGTH OF VOWELS

Vowels are either short or long. Short vowels are **a**, **i**, **u**, and **ṛ**. Long vowels are **ā**, **ī**, **ū**, **e**, and **o**. A long vowel is held for twice as long as a short one.

VOWELS

The English equivalents are approximations.

a as in *but* or *cup*	**ā** as in *father* or *calm*
i as in *sit* or *pick*	**ī** as in *seat* or *clean*
u as in *put* or *pull*	**ū** as in *pool* or *mood*
e as in *save* or *wait*	**o** as in *coat* or *cone*

ṛ is a vowel pronounced with the tip of the tongue bent slightly back toward the roof of the mouth, while making a sound between the **ur** in *curd* and the **ri** in *cricket.*

The next two vowels are diphthongs, combinations of sounds that are made up of two distinct vowels pronounced in rapid succession. Each diphthong, represented by two letters in transliteration, is written as a single letter in the Sanskrit alphabet and has the same length as a long vowel.

ai as in *pie* or *sky*

au as in *town* or *cow*

CONSONANTS

c as in *such,* never as in *cave* or *celery*

s as in *seek* or *sight*

CONSONANTS (continued)

ś	as in *shine* or *shower*
ṣ	is pronounced like **ś**, except that the tip of the tongue is bent slightly back toward the roof of the mouth, as in English *assure.*
t, d, n	are pronounced with the tip of the tongue against the top teeth.
ṭ, ḍ, ṇ	are pronounced with the tip of the tongue bent slightly back to touch the roof of the mouth.
ph	as in *pin* or *uphold,* never as in *photo* or *phase*
th	as in *top* or *hothouse,* never as in *think* or *there*
ṁ	denotes not the consonant *m,* but simply a nasalization of the preceding vowel, as in the three nasal sounds in the French phrase *un grand pont.*
ṅ	as in *ink, ingot,* or *sing*
ñ	as in *bench* or *enjoy*
jñ	as **gny**. Represents a single letter in the Sanskrit alphabet.
r	is a rolled **r**, as in Spanish *para.*
v	is a soft **v** when following a vowel or beginning a word; when following a consonant (as in *tvam*), it is like a **w** but with minimal rounding of the lips.
ḥ	at the end of a line indicates that the previous vowel (or the second vowel in a preceding diphthong) is echoed; for example, *śāntiḥ* is pronounced *śāntihi,* and *durjayaiḥ* is pronounced *durjayaihi.*

When consonants are followed by **h**, as in **bh**, **ph**, **dh**, **gh**, or **ch**, the consonant is aspirated, as in *abhor, uphold, adhere, doghouse,*or *woodchuck.*

A consonant written twice, such as **dd** or **tt**, is pronounced as a single sound and is held twice as long as a single consonant.

Glossary

Transliterations in square brackets are from Sanskrit unless otherwise noted; this may not apply to names of people and deities.

ACTION, ORGANS OF [Sanskrit: *karmendriyas*]
According to traditional Indian philosophy, the five human powers that control the actions of speech, grasping, locomotion, procreation, and excretion.

AGAMA(S) [*āgama*]
Divinely revealed texts, sacred to the Shaivite tradition of India. *See also* SHAIVITE.

ARJUNA [*arjuna*]
One of the warrior heroes in the Indian epic *Mahābhārata*; a disciple of Lord Kṛṣṇa. It was to Arjuna that Kṛṣṇa imparted his teachings in the *Bhagavad-gītā*. *See also* BHAGAVAD-GITA; KRISHNA, LORD.

BHAGAVAD-GITA [*bhagavad-gītā*]
Lit., "song of the Lord." One of the world's treasures of spiritual wisdom, the centerpiece of the Indian epic *Mahābhārata*. In its eighteen chapters, Lord Kṛṣṇa instructs his disciple Arjuna about steady wisdom, meditation, the nature of God, the supreme Self, and spiritual knowledge and practice. *See also* KRISHNA, LORD; SELF.

BISTAMI, HAZRAT BAYAZID [*hazrat bāyazīd bistāmī*]
An ecstatic ninth-century Sūfī saint of northeastern Persia, also known as Abū Yazīd al-Bistāmī; author of many poems that boldly portray the mystic's total absorption in God. *See also* SUFI.

CHITI [fem. = *citi*; masc. = *cit*]
Lit., "Consciousness." The all-pervasive dynamic power of supreme Consciousness that creates, sustains, and dissolves the entire universe; also, the power that conceals and reveals the Truth in human beings. *When capitalized*: The personification of this power as the Goddess, and sometimes more specifically as Kuṇḍalinī Śakti, the power of spiritual evolution in a human being. *See also* CONSCIOUSNESS; KUNDALINI SHAKTI.

CONSCIOUSNESS [Sanskrit: *cit, citi, saṁvit*]
When capitalized: The luminous, self-aware, and creative Reality that is the essential Self of all that exists; a name for God, the Absolute, the supreme Truth. *See also* SELF.

GURU [*guru*]
Lit., "a venerable person, a spiritual preceptor, a teacher." *When capitalized*: A realized Master, a true Guru.

JANAKA, KING [*janaka*]
A royal sage of ancient India who attained liberation through perfect fulfillment of his duties as king, while

remaining completely unattached to the pain and pleasures associated with them.

JNANESHVARI [Marathi: *jñāneśvarī*]
A renowned commentary on the *Bhagavad-gītā*, written in Marathi verse by Jñāneśvar Mahārāj in the late thirteenth century. *See also* BHAGAVAD-GITA; JNANESHVAR MAHARAJ.

JNANESHVAR MAHARAJ [*jñāneśvar mahārāj*]
(1275-1296) The foremost poet-saint of Mahārāṣṭra, also known as Jñānadev. The *Jñāneśvarī*, his commentary in Marathi verse on the *Bhagavad-gītā*, is widely acknowledged as one of the world's greatest spiritual works. *See also* BHAGAVAD-GITA.

KABIR [*kabīr*]
(ca. 1440-1518) A Siddha and devotional poet, who worked as a weaver in Vārāṇasī, India. Said to have been raised in a Muslim family, Kabīr received initiation (*dīkṣā*) from the Guru Rāmānanda of the Hindu tradition, and thereafter continually praised the God beyond form and distinction, who transcends all religions. *See also* GURU; SIDDHA.

KASHMIR SHAIVISM
The nondual Shaivism of medieval Kashmir, a philosophy elaborated in the collective writings of a number of sages from Kashmir for whom the name Śiva denoted the ultimate Reality. These sages, who flourished from the ninth through the twelfth centuries, recognized the entire universe as a manifestation of Śiva's Śakti or divine power. Swami Muktananda found his own experience reflected in the writings of these sages and incorporated many of their core teachings into the philosophical framework of the Siddha Yoga path. *See also* SHAIVISM; SHAKTI; SHIVA, LORD; SIDDHA YOGA.

KRISHNA, LORD [*kṛṣṇa*]
Lit., "dark one." The eighth incarnation of Lord Viṣṇu (a name for the all-pervasive, supreme Reality, the sustainer of the universe), called Kṛṣṇa because of the blue-black color of his skin. *See also* BHAGAVAD-GITA.

KUNDALINI. *See* KUNDALINI SHAKTI.

KUNDALINI SHAKTI [*kuṇḍalinī śakti*]
Lit., "coiled one." The Goddess Kuṇḍalinī; also, the power of spiritual evolution in a human being. The dormant form of this spiritual energy is represented as lying coiled at the base of the spine; when awakened and guided by a Siddha Guru and nourished by the seeker's disciplined effort, this energy brings about purification of the seeker's being at all levels, and leads to the permanent experience of one's divine nature. *See also* GURU; SIDDHA.

MIRABAI [*mīrābāī*]
An early sixteenth-century saint and Rājasthāni princess, who was famous for her poems of devotion to Lord Kṛṣṇa; she was so absorbed in love for Kṛṣṇa that when she was given poison by vindictive relatives, she drank it as nectar and remained unharmed. *See also* KRISHNA, LORD.

NADI [*nāḍī*]
A channel through which the life force is circulated in the human body. In the physical body, *nāḍīs* take the form of blood vessels, nerves, and lymph ducts; in the subtle body, they

constitute a complex system of channels through which the *prāṇa* flows. *See also* PRANA; SUBTLE BODY.

PATANJALI [*patañjali*]
(ca. third century CE) Sage and author of the *Yoga-sūtra*, the authoritative text on one of the six orthodox philosophies of India. *See also* YOGA-SUTRA.

PRANA [*prāṇa*]
The life force; the vital energy within all living things; the vital breath; life.

PRANAYAMA [*prāṇayāma*]
Lit., "restraining the breath." A yogic technique, consisting of systematic regulation and restraint of the breath, which leads to steadiness of mind. It may also occur spontaneously through the power of the awakened Kuṇḍalinī. *See also* KUNDALINI SHAKTI.

PRATYABHIJNA-HRIDAYAM [*pratyabhijñā-hṛdayam*]
Lit., "the heart of recognition." An eleventh-century treatise by Kṣemarāja that expounds on the *pratyabhijñā* (recognition) philosophy of Kashmir Shaivism. It teaches that individuals, having forgotten their true nature, can once again recognize their own Self through divine grace and an experiential understanding of supreme Consciousness as the essence of all creation. *See also* CONSCIOUSNESS; KASHMIR SHAIVISM; SELF.

PURANA(S) [*purāṇa*]
Lit., "ancient." Sacred books of India, containing accounts, stories, legends, and hymns about the creation of the universe, the incarnations of God, the teachings of various deities, and the spiritual legacies of ancient sages and kings.

SADHANA [*sādhanā*]
Leading straight to a goal; a means of accomplishing (something); spiritual practice; worship. The *sādhanā* of Siddha Yoga students, which begins with *śaktipāt* initiation, includes active, disciplined engagement with the essential Siddha Yoga practices of meditation, chanting, *sevā* (selfless service), and *dakṣiṇā* (offering of financial resources), along with focused study and contemplation of the Siddha Yoga teachings. The goal of Siddha Yoga *sādhanā* is the spiritual transformation that leads to liberation. *See also* SIDDHA YOGA.

SAHASRARA [*sahasrāra*]
Lit., "one thousand spokes." The highest spiritual center of the subtle body and the destination of the awakened Kuṇḍalinī; located at the crown of the head, it is often visualized or represented as a lotus with one thousand petals. *See also* KUNDALINI SHAKTI; SUBTLE BODY.

SAMADHI [*samādhi*]
The practice of absorption in the object of meditation; also, the state of meditation in which the meditator is absorbed in the supreme Self. *See also* SELF.

SELF [Sanskrit: *ātman*]
When capitalized: The pure Consciousness that is both the divine core of a human being and the essential nature of all things. *See also* CONSCIOUSNESS.

SHAIVISM
The Indian religious and philosophical traditions that use the name Śiva to denote the ultimate Reality. On the Siddha Yoga path, the term *Shaivism* is generally used to refer to the nondual

Shaivism of Kashmir. *See also* KASHMIR SHAIVISM; SHAIVITE; SHIVA, LORD; SIDDHA YOGA.

SHAIVITE
[*as noun*] One who honors God or the supreme Self in the form of Śiva; one who practices Shaivism; [*as adjective*] of, relating to, or characteristic of Shaivism. *See also* KASHMIR SHAIVISM; SELF; SHAIVISM; SHIVA, LORD.

SHAKTI [*śakti*]
Power, energy, strength. Also, a specific power or energy, such as a power embodied in a particular goddess or within an aspirant. *When capitalized*: The creative power of the divine Absolute, which animates and sustains all forms of creation; often personified as the Goddess, and sometimes more specifically as Kuṇḍalinī Śakti, the power of spiritual evolution in a human being. *See also* KUNDALINI SHAKTI.

SHANKARACHARYA [*śāṅkarācārya*]
A venerated sage of the eighth century, who formalized the Advaita (nondual) school of Vedānta. He established monastic orders in India that exist to this day, including the Sarasvatī order, to which the Siddha Yoga Swamis belong. *See also* SIDDHA YOGA; VEDANTA.

SHIVA, LORD [*śiva*]
Lit., "auspicious." In nondual Shaivism, the transcendent, immanent, and all-pervasive Reality, the one source of all existence. Also, absolute Reality personified as the supreme Deity, Lord Śiva. *See also* KASHMIR SHAIVISM; SHAIVISM.

SHIVA-SUTRA [*śiva-sūtra*]
An important text in the tradition of nondual Shaivism, said to have been revealed to the sage Vasugupta in Kashmir around the middle of the ninth century. The text consists of seventy-seven aphorisms (*sūtras*) conveying profound teachings on the nature of Reality. *See also* KASHMIR SHAIVISM; SHAIVISM.

SIDDHA [*siddha*]
A perfected, fully accomplished, Self-realized yogi; an enlightened yogi who lives in the state of unity consciousness; one whose experience of the Self is uninterrupted and whose identification with the ego has been dissolved. *See also* SELF; YOGI.

SIDDHA YOGA [*siddha yoga*]
The spiritual path taught by Gurumayi Chidvilasananda and her Guru, Swami Muktananda. The journey of the Siddha Yoga path begins with *śaktipāt dīkṣā* (spiritual initiation). Through the grace of the Siddha Yoga Master and the student's own steady, disciplined effort, the journey culminates in the constant recognition of divinity within oneself and within the world. *See also* SADHANA.

SIDDHI [*siddhi*]
Any kind of attainment, but especially a supernatural power.

SO'HAM [*so'ham*]
Lit., "That (*so*) I am (*aham*)." The natural vibration of the Self, which seekers experience within through the Guru's grace, and by which they become aware of their identity with the supreme Self. Also, the mantra formed by the syllables *so* (or *saḥ*) and *ham*, repeated with the breath. Also known as the mantra *haṁsa*. *See also* SELF.

SUBTLE BODY [Sanskrit: *sūkṣma-śarīra*]
The body that is composed of a subtle form of *prāṇa* (vital energy), considered in traditional Indian philosophy to be distinct from the gross or physical body; and which contains the system of energy centers and channels through which Kuṇḍalinī Śakti moves. *See also* KUNDALINI SHAKTI; NADI; PRANA.

SUFI [*sūfī*]
A practitioner of Sūfism, the mystical tradition of Islam characterized by ecstatic devotion to God.

SUNDARDAS [*sundardās*]
(ca. 1596-1689) A poet-saint of Delhi, India, who wrote eloquently about the significance of the spiritual Master and the requirements of discipleship.

TUKARAM MAHARAJ [*tukārām mahārāj*]
(ca. 1608-1650) A poet-saint of Mahārāṣtra, India, who earned his livelihood as a village grocer. After receiving spiritual initiation in a dream, Tukārām wrote thousands of devotional songs (*abhaṅgas*), many of which describe his spiritual experiences and the glory of the divine name.

UPANISHAD(S) [*upaniṣad*]
Lit., "the sitting down near (a teacher)" or "secret doctrine." The group of scriptures that distill the esoteric teachings of the Vedas and are the basis for Vedantic philosophy. Most of the various Upaniṣads illuminate the essential teaching that the individual soul and the Absolute are one. *See also* VEDA(S); VEDANTA.

VEDA(S) [*veda*]
Lit., "knowledge." The earliest scriptural compositions of ancient India, regarded as divinely revealed, eternal wisdom. The four Vedas are, in order of antiquity, the *Ṛg-veda* ("Knowledge of the Hymns"), the *Yajur-veda* ("Knowledge of the Sacrificial Formulas"), the *Sāma-veda* ("Knowledge of the Songs of Praise"), and the *Atharva-veda* ("Knowledge of [Sage] Atharvan").

VEDANTA [*vedānta*]
Lit. "end of the Vedas." One of the six orthodox schools of Indian philosophy; its dominant branch is Advaita ("nondual") Vedānta, which teaches that one supreme Principle of being-Consciousness-bliss (*sac-cid-ānanda*) constitutes the whole of Reality, and that the world of multiplicity is ultimately illusory. *See also* UPANISHAD(S).

YOGA [*yoga*]
Lit., "yoking; joining." A method or set of disciplined spiritual practices (including meditation, mantra repetition, concentration, posture, sense control, and ethical precepts) whose ultimate goal is the constant experience of union with the divine Self. *See also* SELF.

YOGA-SUTRA [*yoga-sūtra*]
(ca. third century CE) A collection of aphorisms, written by the sage Patañjali, that expounds a set of specific and practical methods for the attainment of the goal of yoga, or mental tranquility, when the movement of the mind ceases and the Self rests in its own blissful nature as the witness of the mind. *See also* PATANJALI; SELF; YOGA.

YOGI [masc. = *yogi*; fem. = *yogini*]
One who practices yoga. *See also* YOGA.

Further Reading

Selected Books by SWAMI MUKTANANDA

FROM THE FINITE TO THE INFINITE

As Baba traveled the world, seekers from many countries asked question after question about their spiritual practices. With profound insight and compassionate humor, Baba answered them. This volume contains a wealth of those exchanges, offering readers the opportunity to recognize their own questions and to contemplate Baba's responses.

I AM THAT
The Science of Haṁsa from the Vijñāna Bhairava

In this commentary on verse 24 of the *Vijñāna Bhairava*, a classic text of the nondual Shaivism of Kashmir, Baba teaches about the power of the *haṁsa* mantra. Baba reveals the mystical secrets of this form of mantra repetition and explains how, through dedicated practice, one can become established in the unwavering experience of inner divinity.

PLAY OF CONSCIOUSNESS
A Spiritual Autobiography

This unique spiritual autobiography describes Swami Muktananda's own process of inner transformation under the guidance of his Guru, Bhagavan Nityananda. A rare opportunity to study the first-hand account of a Siddha Master's journey to Self-realization.

RESONATE WITH STILLNESS
Daily Contemplations

In a structure designed for daily study, these passages from the writings of Baba Muktananda and Gurumayi Chidvilasananda support an ongoing practice of focused contemplation.

WHERE ARE YOU GOING?
A Guide to the Spiritual Journey

A lively anecdotal introduction to the teachings of the Siddha Yoga path, this book draws from talks given by Baba in public programs in many different places and times. Answering the question that Baba chose for the title of this book stirs profound contemplation: "Where *am* I going? What *am* I really doing with my life?" This compendium of Baba's teachings covers the stages of the spiritual journey from the first understanding of its purpose to the achievement of its goal: perfect freedom and joy.

Selected Books by
GURUMAYI CHIDVILASANANDA

COURAGE AND CONTENTMENT

Opening with Gurumayi's Message talk for 1997, *Wake Up to Your Inner Courage and Become Steeped in Divine Contentment*, this volume includes eight talks in which Gurumayi unfolds the subtle connections between courage and contentment. To face life's challenges with courage and yet to feel content no matter what happens — this is the fruit of ongoing spiritual practice. It is a fruit, Gurumayi teaches, that ripens with intention, constancy, and patience.

ENTHUSIASM

This volume includes talks that Gurumayi gave on her Message for 1996, *Be Filled with Enthusiasm and Sing God's Glory*. "Seize the opportunity to discover boundless enthusiasm," Gurumayi tells us. "Let the practices of yoga unfold miraculous experiences for you." Gurumayi explores virtues such as patience, forgiveness, gentleness, service, and gratitude — all of which enable us to cultivate our innate enthusiasm and ultimately to perceive God's glory everywhere in every moment of our lives.

MY LORD LOVES A PURE HEART
The Yoga of Divine Virtues

In a series of commentaries on chapter 16 of the *Bhagavad-gītā*, Gurumayi offers precise guidance on how to manifest the magnificent virtues of fearlessness, purity of being, steadfastness, freedom from anger, respect, compassion, humility, and selfless service.

SĀDHANĀ OF THE HEART
Siddha Yoga Messages for the Year

This collection contains the original talks in which Gurumayi presented her Messages for the years 1995 to 1999. For Siddha Yoga students around the world, Gurumayi's Message serves as a focus of contemplation and a source of revelation for that year — and beyond. These Message talks, shining with Gurumayi's wisdom and practical guidance, support a seeker's effort on the journey to the experience of the supreme Heart.

THE YOGA OF DISCIPLINE

By contemplating the talks in this volume, the reader learns how to cultivate yogic discipline and how to apply it to everyday activities. Chapters include Gurumayi's teachings on how to bring yogic discipline to seeing, listening, eating, speaking, and thinking, so that we can "break through boundaries and reach the highest goal."

Book by a Siddha Yoga Teacher

THE SPLENDOR OF RECOGNITION
An Exploration of the Pratyabhijñā-hṛdayam,
a Text on the Ancient Science of the Soul
by Swami Shantananda, with Peggy Bendet

The teachings of the *Pratyabhijñā-hṛdayam*, a text from the tradition of Kashmir Shaivism, explain how all human beings and the entire creation are forms of God and how seekers on the spiritual path can know themselves as God. One important aspect of the philosophy examined in this book is the awakening of Kuṇḍalinī Śakti. Sharing his experiences and wisdom from more than thirty years as a Siddha Yoga student and teacher, Swami Shantananda provides an accessible context for understanding and applying these esoteric teachings.

To learn more about
the Siddha Yoga teachings and practices,
visit the Siddha Yoga path website at:

www.siddhayoga.org

For further information about
SYDA Foundation books
and audio, video, and DVD recordings,
visit the Siddha Yoga Bookstore website at:

www.siddhayogabookstore.org

or call 845-434-2000, extension 1700.

From the United States and Canada,
call toll-free 888-422-3334.